Hours of Boredom, Moments of Terror

Temporal Desynchrony in Military and Security Force Operations

Peter A. Hancock and Gerald P. Krueger

Center for Technology and National Security Policy
National Defense University

October 2010

Peter A. Hancock, Ph.D., is a Provost's Distinguished Research Professor and University Pegasus Professor in the Department of Psychology at the University of Central Florida, Orlando.

Gerald P. Krueger, Ph.D., a retired U.S. Army Colonel, has done significant occupational and preventive medicine research and practical applications work with military forces, emphasizing prediction and measurement of soldier performance in stressful work environments.

Defense & Technology Papers are published by the National Defense University Center for Technology and National Security Policy, Fort Lesley J. McNair, Washington, DC. CTNSP Publications are available at: http://www.ndu.edu/ctnsp/publications.html.

Acknowledgments

This paper is based on Dr. Hancock's presentation at the Human Sciences Research Conference: New Approaches to Warrior Development, convened by the Honorable William A. Navas, Jr., Assistant Secretary of the Navy for Manpower and Reserve Affairs, and held June 13th, 2007, at the National Defense University in Washington DC. Dr. Krueger was the facilitator for that conference. The views expressed here are those of the authors and not necessarily those of any of the named agencies.

Contents

Overview

The "hurry up and wait" phenomenon in many military operations is aptly called "hours of boredom," whereas the transition to meet sudden task demands when combat breaks out is sometimes deemed to consist of "moments of terror." Increasingly, other national security and paramilitary force personnel (e.g., police forces, border patrol, operational intelligence agents) also experience long periods of boredom interspersed with all-out response efforts when the going "gets hot." The authors examine resultant psychological and behavioral implications for combatant and security personnel performance as viewed through application of a traditional *human psychological stress model.* Inadequate recognition of the implications resulting from long lull periods, combat pulses, and the need to recover from stress can lead to dysfunctional soldiering as well as poor individual and small unit performance. Accounting for such time-based transitions in the psychological state of military combatants and security force operators is important in configuring *resilience training* for small group leaders, their personnel, and their organizational units.

Introduction

As we seek to come to terms with the rapidly emerging challenges of military and other national security operations in the new millennium it is crucial to take a careful look at the fundamental characteristics of some of the tasks our deployed personnel are now being asked to perform. This assessment embraces a wide spectrum of requirements, since many former military job elements are now subject to outsourcing. Contemporary national security policies witness deployments of large numbers of State Department, international development agencies, and even Justice Department employees, many of whom carry out a myriad of activities with some of the same military characteristics and accompanying psychological and physiological stressors.[1] Our comments may pertain to other national security forces as well, but here we exemplify our points by referring mostly to the tasks and stresses of military personnel. While not unique to the military, the core security tasks that remain for our professional military have evolved under the driving force of a changing environment, including a broad expansion of defense missions; for example, providing humanitarian assistance, stability and security operations,[2] implementation of new technologies, and emerging forms of conflict such as engaging in asymmetric warfare and counterinsurgency operations.[3] Whereas Krueger[4]

---

[1] Terry Pudas and Catherine Theohary, "Reconsidering the Defense Department Mission," in *Civilian Surge: Key to Complex Operations*, Hans Binnendijk and Patrick M. Cronin eds. (Washington, DC: Center for Technology and National Security Policy, 2008), 39–57.

[2] U.S. Army Combined Arms Center. *Stability Operations: U.S. Army Field Manual 3–07.* (Fort Leavenworth, KS: U.S. Army Combined Army Center, 2008), available at http://fas.org/irp/doddir/army/fm3-07.pdf.

[3] U.S. Army Combined Arms Center and the U.S. Marine Corps Combat Development Command. *Counterinsurgency: U.S. Army Field Manual, FM 3–24* and *U.S. Marine Corps Warfighting Publication MCWP 3-33-5.* (Fort Leavenworth, KS: U.S. Army Combined Arms Center, 2006), available at http://usacac.army.mil/CAC/ Repository/ Materials/COIN-FM3-24.pdf.

[4] Gerald P. Krueger, "Contemporary and future battlefields: Soldier stresses and performance," in *Performance under Stress,* Peter A. Hancock and James L. Szalma eds. (Aldershot, UK: Ashgate Publishing, Ltd., 2008), 19–44.

recently outlined an extensive listing of soldier stresses that impact performance of military personnel on contemporary and future battlefields,[5,6] our central thesis here is that identifiable constants remain in the missions that military and other security force personnel are tasked to accomplish, especially in the *temporal rhythm* of these assignments. Often characterized as "hurry up and wait operations," we term these requirements as "hours of boredom and moments of terror." It is these forms of demand and their effect upon performance and health which form our primary concern. These temporal rhythms are normal and expected in military operations, and are becoming so in other security operations as well. Understood in this light, this article asserts that leaders should, in training, prepare their troops for high levels of cognitive and physiological readiness; they need to anticipate executing operational plans that often require patience and apparent, sometimes boring inactivity that will eventually be followed by sustained maximum performance. This is, in turn, is followed by anticipation of the next activity cycle as pulses in the normal sequence of boredom-terror-boredom—which is the military way of things. Advances in anticipatory strategy can help a variety of professional occupations (e.g., police, emergency response, and other security force workers) whose central temporal characteristics are highly similar to this military challenge.

Hours of Boredom, Moments of Terror

Working environments comprised of long periods of quiescence interrupted by crucial but brief periods of intense activity are by no means confined to military and security operations. Any fireman or emergency service provider will confirm the vast majority of their time is taken up with *waiting* (which is often used as a period of preparation). Professional athletes, professional musicians, actors, and the like engage in extensive preparation time that is then punctuated by short, intense, highly stressful periods of performance demand. Indeed, for some individuals like Olympic sprinters or divers, the actual intervals of performance can be measured in mere fractions of a second while the preparation interval can be assessed in terms of a lifetime.

Military missions lie very much in this realm of temporal desynchrony. Today, modern technology exacerbates the already enormous differences between military training-readiness exercises and actual combat performance. For example, while presumably not bored, modern-day fighter pilots might train for years to engage in aerial combat and then never even see their opponent as they "fire and forget" their weapons beyond the range of normal visual perception. Unmanned aerial vehicle (UAV) operators (pilots) housed thousands of miles from the battle front develop significant levels of boredom while monitoring countless hours of satellite video feed depictions of desert terrain which prove

---

[5] Paul T. Bartone, "Resilience under Military Operational Stress: Can Leaders Influence Hardiness?" *Military Psychology* 18, (2006), S131–S148.

[6] Paul T. Bartone, Charles R. Barry, and Robert E. Armstrong, *To Build Resilience: Leader Influence on Mental Hardiness*, Defense Horizons 69 (Washington, DC: Center for Technology and National Security Policy, 2009).

innocuous most of the time.[7] Soldiers and Marines routinely perform numerous nightly patrol missions for weeks without incident, but then when least expected, they are blasted from their armored vehicles by improvised explosive devices (IEDs) in surprise ambushes. In these terms, "hours of boredom and moments of terror" have evolved into "months of monotony and milliseconds of mayhem."[8]

We clearly need to know more about these transformations from periods of chronic underload to episodes of acute overload. One way to understand such transitions is to appeal to the underlying theory of human stress and performance. Thus, it will come as no surprise that we use the Hancock and Warm[9] model of stress and performance capacity here.

The Importance of Transitions[10]

Before beginning a formal analysis of the psychological and behavioral implications of sudden task demand transitions, we first give a brief précis of the relevant components of the Hancock and Warm[9] model whose central tenets are expressed graphically in figure 1. The Hancock and Warm (psychological and performance) model, more widely known as the extended-U model of stress and performance, can be conceptualized as a series of nested envelopes depicting the limitations of *adaptation* protecting any exposed individual (e.g., a soldier) from the threatening vagaries of the environment surrounding him or her. Implicit in this conception is the notion that the soldier is seeking to achieve some desired optimum state which, being dynamic in nature, is never fully achieved for any extended interval of time. In the center of the illustrated continuum is a "normative zone." This represents a desired state of environmental balance and is equated with complete physiological and psychological adjustment. If the individual is working, then the normative zone is very similar to the notion of a "flow" state,[11] in which the individual seems to anticipate each upcoming requirement sequentially and so appears to effortlessly achieve the goal of the present task. We hypothesize that this state is linked with the psychological phenomenon of *déjà vu* in which events actually seem to reoccur. The temporal basis of this phenomenon has recently been articulated.[12]

---

[7] Mary Cummings, "The Effects of High and Low Workload on Human-System Performance in Decentralized Unmanned Vehicle Control" (presentation made to the National Research Council Committee on Human Systems Integration (CO-HSI), Washington, DC, May 20, 2010).

[8] Peter A. Hancock, "Hours of Boredom, Moments of Terror—or Months of Monotony, Milliseconds of Mayhem" (paper presented at the Ninth International Symposium on Aviation Psychology, Columbus, OH, April 1997).

[9] Peter A. Hancock and Joel S. Warm, "A Dynamic Model of Stress and Sustained Attention," *Human Factors* 31 (1989), 519–537.

[10] In one of his Aubrey-Maturin novels, the author Patrick O'Brian comments "on the stage and waiting for the curtain to go up . . . I wonder whether actions have the same distorted sense of time, a present that advances to be sure, but only like the shadow on a dial imperceptibly, and even then it may go back." Patrick O'Brian, *The Letter of Marque* (New York: W.W. Norton, 1988), 216.

[11] Mihaly Csíkszentmihályi, *Flow: The Psychology of Optimal Experience* (New York: Harper and Row, 1990).

[12] Peter A. Hancock, "The Battle for Time in the Brain," in *Time, Limits and Constraints: The Study of Time XIII*, J.A. Parker, P.A. Harris, and C. Steineck eds. (Leiden, The Netherlands: Koninklijke Brill NV, 2010), 65–88.

As a practical example illustrating the theoretical relationship shown in figure 1, consider the case of combat. The traditional inverted-U view of stress, when applied to performance levels, indicates that individuals under the stress of combat will slowly reduce in their response capacity as the stress increases. But is this true? In general we suggest not. A commonly reported experience is that some individuals fight full out as hard as they can for as long as they can. Others don't fight at all.[13] In the former case, individuals can function at a high level for a surprising length of time. However, when they fail, they tend to fail suddenly and drastically, not in a slow and predictable decline. In general parlance, they "fall off the edge of the table," "reach their tolerance threshold," etc., and their respective commanders must understand and respect when they or their soldiers are approaching their own individual limits, although the exigencies of battle often do not permit immediate exclusion from duty. But these are reactions at the very edge of stress tolerance. To begin understanding such reactions we need to start in the center of the illustration.

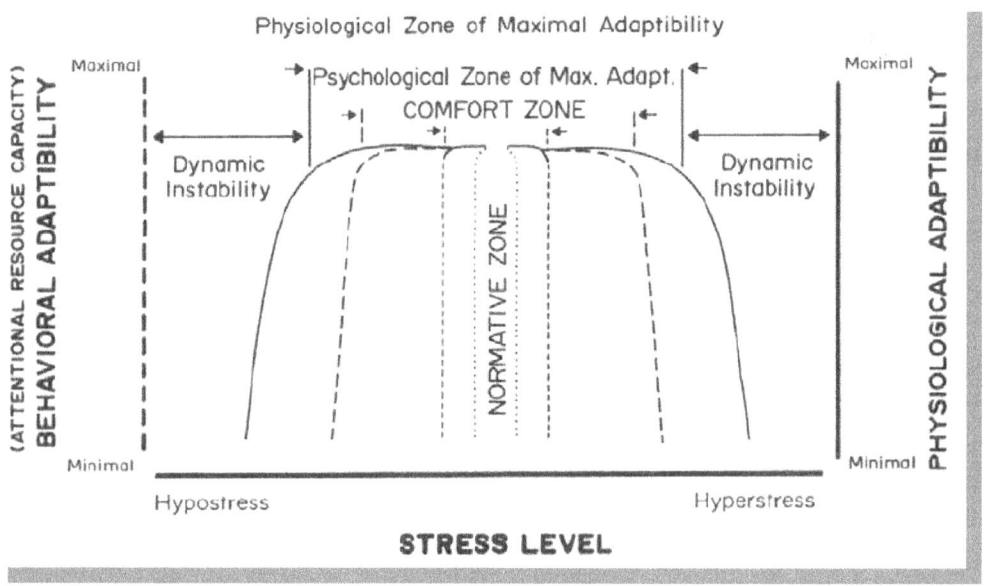

Figure 1: Hancock and Warm Extended-U Stress & Performance Model[14]

Any unanticipated source of disturbance can cause an individual to leave the central, normative zone; a *loss of comfort* is a good indicator of such necessary adjustment. In terms of physiological adaptation, the behavioral indicators of comfort have been neglected for too long as symptoms of stress, especially chronic expressions of stress disturbance. As can be seen in figure 1, each sequential envelope (described by the series

---

[13] S.L.A. Marshall, *Men Against Fire: The Problem of Battle Command in Future War* (New York: William Morrow, 1947).

[14] The extended-U description of capability under stress by Hancock and Warm (1989): The central regions provide an extensive region of relatively stable performance capacity bounded by regions of dynamic instability. Unlike the inverted-U there is no graceful degradation but rather a rapid and distinct precipice of performance failure at the extremes of stress. Changes in capability and response at these thresholds are described in figure 2.

of matched vertical lines around the "comfort zone") actually represents the same fundamental process. The essential process is one of self-survival and it is expressed at a number of differing levels. The two primary levels described in figure 1 are the psychological thresholds describing the brain's appraisal and assessment of the source of threat; the next envelope out is the physiological threshold describing the limits of basic bodily processes. These limits are formally characterized as the progressive failure of *regulated negative feedback*. Such failure is evident as each progressive envelope departs from the flat-topped plateau of the extended-U and begins its descent into degradation of response capacity. Simply put, each expression of response degradation represents a progressively more gross process, starting with those related to achieving goal states and ending up with those that serve solely to preserve life. The characteristic leitmotif of failure is not a slow, graceful degradation of capacity, but a sudden falling "over the edge" of regulatory capacity. Tasks of progressively greater difficulty prove more vulnerable to the same level of stress. Thus, although there are only a limited number of 'envelopes' illustrated, a whole series of such envelopes of success and failure are embedded in the model, and the transition between stable and failing states under any specific stress is contingent upon the demands placed by the task.

A simple physical analogy may help here. A soldier carrying 30 lbs at 50% VO_2Max[15] will last a certain time before experiencing the onset of performance failure. A soldier carrying 60 lbs will last a much shorter time (e.g., the envelope is tighter toward the center of the illustration). A soldier carrying 120 lbs will be very limited in performance capacity. These are simple physiological loads. However, they represent direct analogies in psychological dimensions of task demand. Thus a soldier asked to remember 5 random numbers will be able to perform this quite well under stress but a soldier asked to remember 15 random numbers will be much more vulnerable to that same level of stress. Of course, memory is only one of the psychological capacities that challenge our soldiers and other dimensions of performance such as multiple tasking will prove even more vulnerable. Thus, one primary purpose of technology is to support the soldier, and so alleviate stress-related performance degradation by supporting their task response capacities. This is especially true in stressful conditions so technology that is not user-friendly but actually adds to the demands placed upon the soldier is actually a double disservice to that individual.

The time scale of these various actions also very much depends upon the nature of the disturbance affecting the soldier. In our present case, we evaluate the effects of both *prolonged boredom* and sudden extreme *demand for immediate action* and the *transition* between these two states.

Bartone[5,6] identifies six of the most common soldier stressors in military operations as isolation, ambiguity, powerlessness, boredom (alienation), danger (threat), and workload. Examples of boredom include long periods or repetitive work activities without variety, lack of work that can be construed as meaningful or important, with the overall mission or purpose not understood as being important, and having few options for play and

---

[15] VO_2Max = the respiratory measure of a person's maximum capability for physical energy expenditure—a useful measure of one's state of physical fitness.

entertainment. A key issue influencing the impact of any stress is one's actual and/or perceived level of control over the sources that represent the appraised stress (in some regards, powerlessness). Individuals can tolerate a great deal of stress if they believe they can exercise a moderating influence over it. Conversely, even small levels of stress, if they are unalterable by the actions of the individual, can prove extremely deleterious.

Historically, in the military case, strategic decisions (e.g., deployment patterns) are largely made elsewhere at a higher level of command, not at the soldier level. In contrast, however, modern military forces have been consistently and significantly moving toward delegation of tactical authority. Employing advances in electronics, network-centric communication systems, and individual battlefield computers provides linked, but distributed communications from small teams in "frontline foxholes" to the senior generals in charge, enabling rapid decisionmaking by warfighters at the farthest forward echelon of command.[16,17] Thus, compared to forces two to three generations ago, lower level personnel in contemporary forces have a much greater degree of influence on their own immediate activities. This is expressed in General Charles Krulak's notion of the *Strategic Corporal* wherein even Marines at the first level of command (squad or platoon level) are occasionally expected to engage in rapid, sequential decisionmaking for which the outcomes may have international repercussions.[18] This dispersed autonomy has a beneficial effect on acute stress since the control that it gives the individual ameliorates some of the stress each person experiences, but it still leaves the hours of boredom as a persistent issue.

One of the universal attributes of boredom and underload is that people often don't see "the quiet time" as an issue of stress—that is, waiting for the next sequential event and how that, in effect, interrupts the flow state. On the surface it appears that the individual is doing almost nothing. Unless they are of an ardent "type A" character, then doing 'nothing' appears to be rather acceptable. Indeed, doing nothing is often what we aspire to do on a 'vacation,' and vacations are viewed as a good thing—at least for a while. However, as many retired people find to their considerable stress, having nothing to do for an extended time can be deleterious to one's health. Extended periods of enforced quiescence, especially to normally active people, can represent almost intolerable conditions that strongly interfere with normal cognitive functioning, as extensive literature on sensory and perceptual deprivation and its linkage to prolonged torture

---

[16] David S. Alberts and Richard E. Hayes, *Power to the Edge: Command, Control in the Information Age* (Washington, DC: Command and Control Research Program, Center for Advanced Concepts and Technology, 2003).
[17] Gerald P. Krueger and Louis E. Banderet, "Implications for Studying Team Cognition and Team Performance in Network-Centric Warfare Paradigms," *Aviation, Space, and Environmental Medicine* 78, no. 5 (2007), Section II, B58–B62.
[18] Charles C. Krulak, "The Strategic Corporal: Leadership in the Three Block War," *Marines Corps Gazette* 83 (1999), 18–22.

illustrates.[19,20] Thus our brains are naturally active, and preventing them from engaging in their normal level of activity can be highly damaging.

In combat deployments wherein actual fighting occurs intermittently in pulses and cycles, small unit military leaders often report their leadership challenges include a fair amount of *"boredom, fighting complacency, and maintaining motivation of their troops."* Such concerns are illustrated in the following comments extracted from U.S. Army after action reports:

- "Maintaining morale in my platoon has become a demanding leadership challenge. This is because of the monotony of patrolling with no enemy contact. Soldiers feeling they are not accomplishing anything out in a sector also brings morale down." Chris F., Armor Officer.
- "Fighting complacency, maintaining motivation, and remaining disciplined. This is a battle we fight every day from both ends—platoon as well as higher echelons of command. Defining a purpose for our missions, being prepared at all times for any situation, and staying motivated and transferring that attitude to the platoon." Austin F.J., Infantry Officer.
- "Keeping men focused on the mission while staying in static positions, even upholding basic soldier standards." Erich R., Infantry Officer.
- "Maintaining intensity during a low-intensity conflict with an accelerated battle rhythm." Quinn R., Field Artillery Officer.
- "Keeping my soldier focus and bearing under fire when we were recovering some of our own dead and wounded." Erik K., Infantry Officer.

The above comments[21] confirm that the issues outlined are not merely academic concerns but rather are the direct everyday challenges that face present officers and troops in the field.

These hours, days, weeks, even months of boredom can represent cumulative stress which can result in very adverse effects on both health and performance.[5,22,23,24] However, in the military, such relative inactivity occurs against a background understanding that, at any moment, maximal effort may well be required on occasions

---

[19] John P. Zubek, ed., *Sensory Deprivation: Fifteen Years of Research* (New York: Appleton-Century-Crofts, 1969).

[20] Valtin, "Heart of darkness: Sensory deprivation and U.S. torture—where from here?" Daily KOS Blog, comment posted May 9, 2007, available at <http://www.dailykos.com/story/2007/5/9/234216/8201>.

[21] Interview comments about soldier boredom extracted from Center for Army Lessons Learned After Action Reviews from Small Unit Leaders Following Military Deployment to Conflicts in the Middle East, (2006). Acquired from Department of Behavioral Sciences and Leadership at the U.S. Military Academy at West Point, NY.

[22] Donald O. Hebb, "Drives and the Conceptual Nervous System," *Psychological Review* 62 (1955), 243–254.

[23] Philip Solomon, Herbert Leiderman, Jack Mendelson, and Donald Wexler, "Sensory Deprivation: A Review," *American Journal of Psychiatry* 114 (1957), 357.

[24] S. Weinstein, L. Fisher, M. Richlin, and M. Weisinger, "Bibliography of Sensory and Perceptual Deprivation, Isolation, and Related Areas," *Perceptual and Motor Skills* 26 (1968), 11–19.

when the bullets start to fly. Military personnel compensate for intervals of boredom by participating in training, maintenance, additional activities and duties, and using modern electronic access to make contact with home and family. Maintaining such continuous activity levels may even lead to over-compensation resulting in mental fatigue and exhaustion. Keeping a time-related activity balance on active deployed military duty is a difficult challenge. If periods of boredom are a problem, so are the sudden transitions to combat action. As anyone who has received a sudden fright knows, the body reacts strongly to the perception of immediate threat.[25] Various physiological and neurological reactions are put in motion to permit the body to respond to upcoming, perceived challenges. Such global alerting effects have a cost in respect to bodily capacity. They can be easily tolerated on a relatively infrequent basis, and if our normal life becomes too mundane, we even seek to stimulate ourselves in some fashion (e.g., purposefully watching scary movies).

However, repeatedly being subjected to these sudden transitions from boredom to ultimate action can have damaging long-term physiological and psychological effects. These effects have been noted in arousal-based bodily systems (e.g., hormonal, circulatory). What we have much less knowledge and understanding of is how these repeated incidents of threat affect cognitive functioning. Like all other aspects of stress, we expect that high frequencies of sudden transition from one state to the other and perhaps back again will have a harmful influence. As well as stress-based concerns, there are many performance-based issues associated with sudden task-load transitions.[26] In this case, what we hypothesize refers to the "shoulders" or edges of failure as expressed by the down slope drop off curves in figure 1 (Hancock and Warm's stress model[9]). Component elements of these shoulders are represented in particular detail in figure 2. Capacities become unstable in these regions, exhibiting decreases in mean level of performance accompanied by increases in response variability. Since the first form of decrease reflects in the first "moment"[27] of response distributions (e.g., the mean level of response) and the second form of symptom of degradation is reflected in the second "moment" (e.g., the variability of an individual's response), the combined effect is a systematic influence on the coefficient of variation (COV). This is because the coefficient of variation is derived from the division of the standard deviation (variability) score by the mean value of the current level of performance. Thus, systematic changes in COV over time are those which induce the chronic damage and represent the major effect of repeated transitions.

This phase transition (e.g., from boredom to immediate action) is very much related to the use of information within the individual person. In general, both physiological and psychological processes (which we contend are largely reflections of the same general use of energetic information) are dominated by the dampening effects of negative feedback. As the thermostat on the wall acts to keep room temperature at acceptable

---

[25] Hans Selye, *The Stress of Life* (New York: McGraw-Hill, 1976).

[26] Beverly M. Huey and Christopher D. Wickens, *Workload Transition: Implications for Individual and Team Performance* (Washington, DC: National Academy Press, 1993).

[27] Here, "moment" refers to the formal way of describing distributions. It does not mean the moment in time.

levels, so negative feedback loops in the body look to counteract the effects of stresses encountered in the environment. These notions reflect the classic insights of Claude Bernard, Walter Cannon, and other early luminaries, in what was termed the concept of homeostasis.[28] This use of regulatory feedback is clearly advisable for any individual hoping to survive and prosper in an uncertain environment. In essence, this is a conservative but still adaptive strategy.

Embedded within this general approach is the use of *feed-forward* or anticipatory mechanisms. Imagine that you are going out on a mission. It is a good idea to plan that mission first, and to generate a list of the resources one might need and then collect these prior to departure. These are direct examples of anticipatory (or feed-forward), mechanisms which are embedded in bodily response. Arguably, it is the superior level of this capacity to anticipate the future in detail that offsets human beings from the rest of the animal kingdom. Largely predicated upon past experience, it is vital for the growth of our adaptive capacity that the individual anticipate the coming conditions, at least to some degree.[12] Each of these strategies, negative feedback and positive feed-forward serve the individual well in circumstances in which conditions are largely anticipatable, or more colloquially, "normal."

However, axiomatically normal anticipation does not work well in conditions that are exceptional. Consequently, such strategies are less advisable, especially in very exceptional circumstances. Similarly, the dampening of negative feedback can inhibit the immediate use of full capacities in just those moments where they are needed to survive. In the transition phase identified in figure 2 (see bold bracket), we see a representation of the individual (in this case the human operator) transferring from the everyday negative feedback and positive feed-forward, as shown by the phase transition region. It is this manifest variation in someone's normal behavior that begins to indicate the onset of possible failure. These later processes are largely emergency, reactive responses and may well be adapted to sudden emergency conditions; but they are abrasive and chronically damaging to the individual and are only enacted because they are preferable to extinction. That these emergency responses are sometimes inappropriate in a modern world, or that they are damaging if they persist across longer intervals of time, represents some of the stress problems faced by military or other security personnel in harm's way.

---

[28] Walter B. Cannon, *The Wisdom of the Body* (New York: W.W. Norton, 1932).

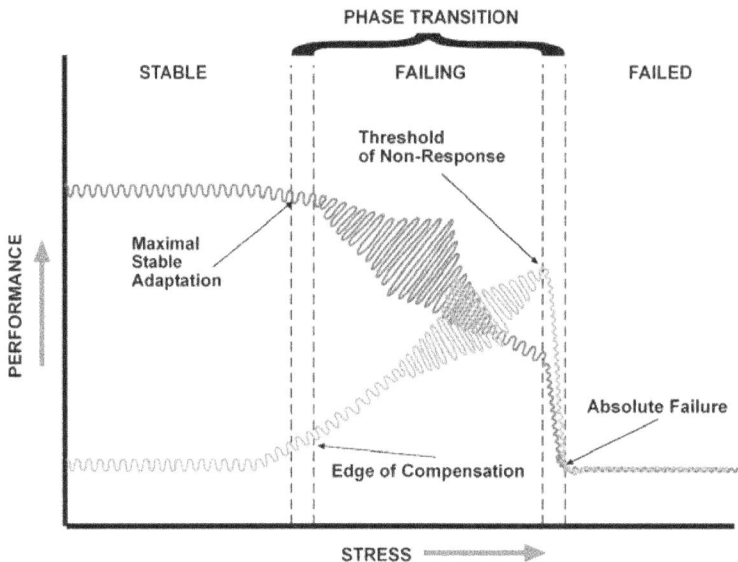

Figure 2: Hancock and Warm Phase Transition toward Failure at the Edge of Adaptability[29]

Here, stress is seen as that influence that pulls the individual away from longer-range planning activities and stable, error-correction regulation (e.g., a military intelligence officer anticipating and plotting likely responses of friendly forces to enemy activities) toward reactive responses that are largely dictated by the immediate and momentary vagaries of the environment around them (e.g., responses to artillery or ambush attack). From a reasoning, planning person, largely in control of his or her situation, the individual becomes almost like a puppet, dancing to the immediate demands of the world directly around them. It is little wonder then that control and perceived control are such important mediators of stress effects.[30,31] The exhaustion expressed in the latter phases of Selye's physiological stress model derives because the individual is constantly on watch against the perceived imminent threat. More formally, stress acts to shrink the future anticipative element of perception and action.[32,33] This very much implies that stress acts as the primary agent of evolutionary adaptation and that the failure of adaptation under

---

[29] Performance capacity failure at the edge of adaptability. The extended-U description indicates that performance remains relatively stable for extensive ranges of stress (expressed at the left of the illustration and extending well out to the left as shown in figure 1). As failure begins to be expressed, we see an increase in the variability of speed of response (upper line) and error of response (lower line). These are symptoms of a phase transition between feed-forward and feed-back–based response strategies. These are the first symptoms of incipient failure.

[30] Robert A. Karasek, "Job Demands, Job Decision Latitude and Mental Strain: Implications for Job Redesign," *Administrative Science Quarterly* 24 (1979), 285–306.

[31] Robert A. Karasek and Tores Theorell, *Healthy Work: Stress, Productivity and the Reconstruction of Working Life* (New York: Basic Books, 1990).

[32] Peter A. Hancock and Mark H. Chignell, "On Human Factors," in *The Ecology of Human-Machine Systems: I. Global Perspectives,* J. Flach, Peter A. Hancock, Jeffrey K. Caird and Kim Vicente, eds. (Mahwah, NJ: Erlbaum Associates, 1995).

[33] Nelville Moray and Peter A. Hancock, "Minkowski Spaces as Models of Human-Machine Communication," *Theoretical Issues in Ergonomics Science* 10, no. 4 (2008), 315–334.

the driving force of stress is not simply an influence on the evolution of a particular species, but has its most direct and immediate effects on the exposed individual.

In human beings this is inevitably a complex process because of our strong social nature. Military personnel benefit from "shared stress buffering" in their social groups represented by teams, crews, patrols, squads, units, groups, battalions, and so on. All take extensive advantage of the fact that the group is much more resilient than the equivalent number of isolated individuals. However, just as the capacity limit envelopes expressed in the Hancock and Warm stress model (figure 1) are each expressions of sequential limits of the same general sort, so too the group will also eventually fail if the stress is extreme enough or persists for a long enough interval. In examining current, repeated deployment practices of Western forces in the Mideast conflicts, it is possible we are starting to see the symptoms of such group failure.

Having dealt with chronic boredom and underload and the transition between states of boredom and states of emergency, we now focus specifically on the breakdown of performance during the "moments of terror." Often, combat missions require the individual to do something that is highly paradoxical. Military actions ask that for an expressed "higher" purpose, individuals expose themselves to significant threats which are known to cause either injury or fatality. A frank cognitive appraisal of such a proposition shows just how curious this is. While it is true that numerous nonmilitary people face fatal circumstances on many occasions (perhaps excepting firemen and policemen), they rarely do so on a purely voluntary basis. What this means is that every combat mission possesses elements of unique stress which occur before, during, and after events. This tripartite differentiation is very much representative of Haddon's matrix[34] of stress as viewed over phased temporal flow, an example of the structure of which is presented in table 1.

Using Haddon's simple matrix of stress by temporal flow we can follow the experience of an individual exposed to sudden emergency conditions. Haddon identifies three temporal phases (table 1, vertical axis), logically enough—before, during, and after significant events, (labeled as pre-event, event, and post-event) and four components of that temporal flow (on the horizontal axis labeled as host, agent, physical environment, and social environment). The host in this case is the military Serviceperson (Soldier, Marine), and the agent is the source of threat (e.g., enemy combatants). The physical environment is that which surrounds the Serviceperson (e.g., high altitude mountainous terrain), while the social environment is composed of interactions with all other pertinent individuals (e.g., peers, leaders, subordinates, indigenous personnel in peace-keeping). In the military, Soldiers (the host) *pre-plan* as much as possible in the pre-event phase, considering the sources of threat, the conditions in which the action will occur and who is likely to be there, whether friends, foes, or neutrals. While the action (significant *event*) is in progress these are also the primary sources of concern, those which serve to focus the conduct of any after-action review, the *post-event phase.*

---

[34] William Haddon, Jr., "On the Escape of Tigers: An Ecologic Note," *American Journal of Public Health,* 60, no. 12, (1970), 2229–2234.

Table 1: William Haddon's Matrix of Stress by Phased Temporal Flow[35]

	Host (e.g. soldier)	Agent (e.g. source of threat)	Physical Environment (e.g. desert, mountains, forest, etc.)	Social Environment (e.g. interactions with others)
PHASE				
Pre-Event (e.g. planning)				
Event				
Post-Event (e.g. after action review)				

Combat and conflict situations often can be difficult to comprehend during action because of the spatial and temporal distortions of perception that accompany high-stress events.[36] Haddon's matrix offers a descriptive approach, which helps us to structure our understanding of events that permit the accuracy and anchor-effects that pre- and post-event evaluations encourage. Since "moments of terror" are fleeting yet so crucially important, any structure that can be brought to these life-changing moments is vital. In a matter of milliseconds, lives can be altered forever. What we now begin to realize is that the self-same effects of these moments of terror can be transmitted about as effectively by the many hours of boredom, and the repeated transitions between these two states of boredom and terror. One important behavioral indication of these effects is noted in the rising incidence of post-traumatic stress disorder among previously deployed military personnel.

Post-Traumatic Stress Disorder

As Bartone[5] points out, many combatants suffer physical and mental health decrements following exposure to stress, while many others show remarkable resilience, remaining healthy despite high stress levels, even when working in the same military unit. One of the most critical concerns of the military, especially for Army and Marine ground forces, is the issue of post-traumatic stress disorder (PTSD). In some ways, it is not appropriate to label this a "disorder," because post-traumatic stress states are perfectly reasonable systemic reactions to the perfectly unreasonable levels of stress and strain encountered by

---

[35] Haddon's (1970) Matrix. On the vertical axis are the three components of temporal flow. On the horizontal axis there are four forms of entity experiencing this flow. These are first, the Host represents the person at risk of damage. The second element is the Agent, the energy type which poses the threat, e.g., kinetic energy from weapons. The third element is the Physical Environment, the setting in which the threats occur. Lastly is the Social Environment referring to the norms and practices the particular culture expects and imposes on Hosts.

[36] Peter A. Hancock and Jeanie L. Weaver, "On Time Distortions under Stress," *Theoretical Issues in Ergonomics Science* 6, no. 2 (2005), 193–211.

our troops. In our minds, PTSD is often correlated with particular "spectacular events."[37] Given our Western view of causation, this is a common and reasonable way to understand the phenomenon. Such events may be the psychological trauma caused by witnessing sudden death or injury, or may be from the physical trauma of repeated "shell-shock" stressors such as incoming artillery blast over-pressures.[38] PTSD is a complex issue since it also involves the prior experiences of the individual, his/her immediate exposure to particular circumstances, and subsequent experiences both within the military following deployment and extending to experiences after returning from dangerous overseas deployments.[39]

PTSD can be represented as a chronic effect of prolonged stress over which one has little to no control. Such maladaptive conditions involve continuous threat of traumatic fatality and exposure to conditions and events for which an individual is unprepared. Military combat and its sequelae often expose individuals to events for which no normal human being can be fully prepared[40] (see reported experiences in Iraq;[41] and see embedded journalist Sebastian Junger's vivid examples of endless anticipation of battle in front line infantry operations in Afghanistan[42]). It is perhaps one of the great ironies of all military engagements that even the victors have to live with the consequences of their actions, for example killing one's adversaries,[43,44] consequences that can prove morally and psychologically corrosive over the years to follow. In this way, the stress of combat affects not only the exposed individuals but society in general.

As any nation increases its standard of living and the associated expectations of its citizens, those who volunteer or are selected for military service and national security jobs will become progressively less adapted to the rigors and experiences of war. This, for example, was why Thomas More advocated that "utopians" use mercenaries for their wars. Despite all the blather about video-game preparation of future soldiers, the higher the level of education that is provided for a nation's citizens the more the antipathy for the actual process of war. At least hopefully this is true. Thus, we have an ever-growing moral obligation to those who fight the nation's battles in helping to readjust after their

---

[37] Matthew J. Friedman, Terence M. Keane, and Patricia A. Resick, eds., *Handbook of PTSD: Science and Practice* (New York: Guilford Press, 2007).

[38] David Marlowe, "The Human Dimension of Battle and Combat Breakdown," in *Military Psychiatry: A Comparative Perspective*, ed. R.A. Gabriel (New York: Greenwood Press, 1986), 7–24.

[39] Rick L. Campise, Schuyler K. Geller, and Mary E. Campise, "Combat Stress," in *Military Psychology: Clinical and Operational Applications,* Carrie H. Kennedy and Eric A. Zillmer, eds. (New York: Guilford Press, 2006), 215–240.

[40] Daryl S. Paulson and Stanley Krippner, *Haunted by Combat: Understanding PTSD in War Veterans Including Women, Reservists, and Those Coming Back from Iraq* (Westport, CT: Praeger Security International, 2007).

[41] J.L. Merlo, Michael M. Szalma, and Peter A. Hancock, "Stress and Performance: Some Experiences from Iraq," in *Performance under Stress,* Peter A. Hancock and James L. Szalma, eds. (Aldershot, UK: Ashgate Publishing, Ltd., 2008), 359–379.

[42] Sebastian Junger, *War* (New York, NY: Hachette Book Group, Inc., Grand Central Publishing, 2010).

[43] David A. Grossman, *On Killing: The Psychological Cost of Learning to Kill in War and Society* (New York: Little-Brown, 1995).

[44] David A. Grossman and Loren W. Christensen, *On Combat: The Psychology of Deadly Conflict in War and Peace* (Belleville, IL: PPCT Research Publications, 2004).

military service is complete. In the Western world, our naïve expectation is that all can be repaired or regenerated as it was before such exposure. This is incorrect. Some individuals who serve and experience the extreme stresses of war will never fully recover. Given the advances in biocybernetics and prosthetics, it may well be that the physical injuries of combat will eventually be more easily accommodated than the psychological damage. The former is more directly observable, the latter more insidious.

Summary and Recommendations

We have highlighted here some of the issues of sudden psychological and physiological transitions between temporal periods of boredom and overloading moments (of terror) as well as the potential for performance degradation and stress-related health problems that they engender. While there is not much research published on *boredom* per se, a recent book by two Norwegian professors[45] asserts that wars consist of 95% boredom and 5% horror, and that boredom imparts certain demands on individual workers who endure it. Supervisors who ignore boredom exhibit poor leadership. In its simplest form, boredom can endanger operations, even military ventures, as it may even lead to tactical and strategic failures at a later time.

The obvious question is—what can we advise military commanders or leaders and supervisors of security force personnel to do about this?

Recommendations for Commanders, Leaders, and Supervisors

- *Recognize rhythms in human activity.* Leaders must first recognize that the rhythms in human activity (including military and security force activities) are natural and inherent expressions of human behavior. In actual fact, such temporal-based rhythms are most helpful in regulating and modulating both cognitive and physical load. What we need to ensure is that the changes from one phase to another are not so abrupt as to be damaging to workers (e.g., soldiers, security personnel). Practical strategies to elongate the transition interval by minimizing the hours of boredom should prove to be most useful to help dilute the phase shift to moments of terror. Practice in training activities, readiness exercises, and preparation for emergency calls-to-action can serve this function.
- *Spread out cognitive task demands.* Similarly, shifting some of the cognitive load of sudden response to the intervals of quiescence can reduce the stress on pressured personnel. This strategy has already been enacted in the design and operation of complex human-machine systems; such 'load-leveling' operations are referred to as "adaptive allocation." Approaches that focus on the minimization of large fluctuations of imposed task-demand often use pre-programmed responses to adjust the imposed load when some particular load threshold has been crossed.[46,47,48,49]

---

[45] Bard Maeland and Paul Otto Brunstad, *Enduring Military Boredom: From 1750 to the Present* (Hampshire, UK: Palgrave Macmillian, 2010).

[46] Peter A. Hancock, "On the process of automation transition in multi-task human-machine systems," Transaction of the IEEE on Systems, Man, and Cybernetics, *Part A: Humans and Systems* 37, no. 4 (2007), 586–598.

These self-same principles can be applied at the individual or group level using both technical and planning support to distribute the imposed operational load—and so dissolve the inherent stress of the sudden call to action during the moments of terror.

- *Acknowledge physiological rhythms.* Just as combatant leaders understand that battles are fought in pulses, they should understand some of the normal human bodily and biological rhythms as well. As mentioned earlier, human beings naturally oscillate in their various physiological capacities, and among these forms of oscillation, circadian physiological rhythms are perhaps the most well known.[50] However, there also are ultradian and infradian rhythms having frequencies which are either faster or slower than the circadian change across the 24-hour interval. Amongst these, the basic rest-activity cycle shows that continuous activity in the 2–3 hour range is well tolerated but prolonged activities which exceed a period of 4 hours in duration tend to prove more problematic. Well-planned use of work-rest breaks, and changing or alternating activities every couple of hours can help to break up monotony.

- *Plan for adequate rest and sleep.* Commanders and leaders must recognize the many human factors involved in *sustained and/or continuous operations* and the inherent performance implications attached to working for extensively long hours without adequate sleep. Leaders need to assign sufficient personnel staffing in the workplace for sustaining operations; design and implement appropriate work-rest scheduling for the mission; and recognize the need and then develop and adhere to individual and work-unit sleep discipline policies and practices. These are outlined by Krueger.[51,52] The degree of stress imposed in sustained or continuous around-the-clock operations is of course contingent upon what the individuals are being asked to do for those extended intervals. Dull, repetitive work can lead to boredom, inattention, compromised vigilance, missed signals, etc. Often, it is the boring and supposedly undemanding tasks like watch-keeping that actually impose significant levels of stress.[9] It is also often the underload element, combined with the knowledge that failure in that element can lead to serious if not fatal consequences for oneself and one's colleagues, that imposes the greatest long-term sources of stress. This is all the more insidious since this stress remains hidden because these tasks "appear" to be so simple and apparently undemanding.

---

[47] Peter A. Hancock and Mark H. Chignell, "Adaptive Control in Human-Machine Systems," in *Human Factors Psychology*, ed. Peter A. Hancock (Amsterdam: North-Holland, 1987), 305–345.

[48] Raja Parasuraman and M. Mouloua, eds., *Automation and Human Performance: Theory and Applications* (Hillsdale, N.J.: Erlbaum Associates, 1996).

[49] Raja Parasuraman and Peter A. Hancock, "Mitigating the adverse effects of workload, stress and fatigue with adaptive automation," in *Performance Under Stress*, Peter A. Hancock and James L. Szalma, eds. (Aldershot, UK: Ashgate Publishing, Ltd, 2008), 45–57.

[50] Wilse B. Webb, ed., *Biological Rhythms, Sleep and Performance* (Chichester, UK: Wiley and Sons, 1982).

[51] Gerald P. Krueger, "Sustained Work, Fatigue, Sleep Loss and Performance: A Review of the Issues," *Work and Stress* 3, no. 2 (1989), 129–141.

[52] Gerald P. Krueger, "Sustained Military Performance in Continuous Operations: Combatant Fatigue, Rest and Sleep Needs," in *Handbook of Military Psychology*, Rueven Gal and A. David Mangelsdorff, eds. (Chichester, UK: John Wiley and Sons, 1991), 255–277.

- *Train to anticipate both hours of boredom and moments of terror*. Perhaps the most helpful approach military commanders and civilian security force supervisors can take in preparing their personnel for hours of boredom and moments of terror is to offer practice in realistic training that mimics actual anticipated operations as close as possible. Troops naturally deal with the stresses of combat more successfully if they are trained to handle it.[4] In developing "stress hardiness," exposing workers to "stress training scenarios" incorporating the kinds of traumas as well as the periods of boredom they likely will face in actual war or security operations is deemed helpful.[6,53] As a practical matter, repetitive practice and rehearsal can fill some of the unending hours of boredom while readily addressing the sudden ramp up in demand that the call-to-action imposes. However, like all things, if overused, the practice (rehearsal) strategy can itself become a rote burden which annoys and frustrates personnel instead of acting as a source of stress mitigation. In training or preparation for deployment it would be helpful to educate soldiers/security workers about what to expect as the insidious effects of "hours of boredom."

- *Anticipate future technological assists in cognitive assessment*. In a classic human engineering approach, the high demands of many emergency responses can be diminished by transferring some workload to technological support systems (e.g., through application of augmented cognition technologies[54]). This strategy leaves the human responders free to answer the case-specific requirements of particular, unique incidents. Here, it would be of great help for a military commander or a security force director to have some on-line assessment of the cognitive and physiological state of readiness of the individuals under his or her command. This stress-level metric could guide decisions as to immediate response as well as an assessment of more long-term chronic exposure to stress of his or her troops/workers which could be useful in mitigating post-deployment problems. Largely composed of ongoing physiological and cognitive measures, an individual's personal historic profile (prior experiences) could also be factored into the assessment. Although generally useful to assess the readiness of personnel, such information cannot change the fundamental nature of conflict and thus such proposals remain suggestions for consideration and research rather than hard and fast algorithms for stress response.

Concluding Notes

The "hurry up and wait" aspect of military operations, involving long periods of boredom, has been around as long as warfare itself. Today's national security force personnel experience many similarities in their work (e.g., border patrol watch-keeping is not unlike some boring military operations). It is intrinsic to all human warfare that periods of lassitude and inactivity frame the incidence of actual combat. Battles are said to be fought in pulses, partly due to the necessity of moving troops and logistical supplies

---

[53] James E. Driskell, Eduardo Salas, John H. Johnston, and Terry N. Wollert, "Stress exposure training: An Event-Based Approach," in *Performance under Stress*, Peter A. Hancock and James L. Szalma, eds. (Aldershot, UK: Ashgate Publishing, Ltd., 2008), 271–287.

[54] Dylan D. Schmorrow and Kay M. Stanney, eds., *Augmented Cognition: A Practitioner's Guide* (Santa Monica, CA: Human Factors and Ergonomics Society, 2008).

over the geography of the battlefield. Such periods are commonly used for varying forms of preparation, but the waiting time cannot always be fully occupied by logistical preparation, maintenance, and rehearsal activities. Then one of two things happens. The first is that the preparation becomes the "norm" and the fighting force is blunted in proportion, or the alternative is that soldiers or other workers get "bored" and seek other outlets for their energies, not all of them productive or contributory to order.[37] Neither is conducive to maximal preparedness. In some generations, when all-out international conflict is expected but never actually occurs, this can lead to whole generations who prepare for combat but never actually engage in it. In other generations, it can lead to almost permanent deployment as subcritical skirmishes predominate in an insurgency-based action such as currently exists in Iraq and Afghanistan. It is not lost on us that each of these conditions is representative of Selye's original conception of stress stages here.

It would be nice to be able to provide a simple formula that could be followed to dismiss these effects of maladapted temporal rhythms. However, the constraints of conflict and sustained security operations make this unlikely. Rather, the answer lies in familiarizing workers (troops or other security personnel) with these demands of temporal transition both in basic and advanced training. This is difficult since the "adrenaline rush" of real operations is never quite replicated in exercises or simulations and it is the very stimulus of being thrust into immediate action scenarios which permits troops to perform under extended high demand in the first place. Practice at varying the levels of cognitive demand placed on active workers, finding meaningful activities for mission "down times" and emphasizing the importance of variations in activity during off-duty hours can all help mitigate the impact of these sudden and demanding transitions in activity level. With the advent of advanced technology and automation, it is possible to conduct some missions in Afghanistan from control centers resident in the United States.[7] The notion of an automated and technological war might seem farfetched at present, and is far from the experience of combat troops on the ground. Thus, humans are still the central elements in current military and security-based operations, and the best policy for any commander or supervisor is to look after those human resources to the best of his/her ability. This means planning the temporal nature of the deployment experience is an important but as yet not fully resolved issue.